To Fern!
Best wishes
Yours self care
Pat Sayers
11/2/84

SELF-CARE DEFICIT THEORY OF NURSING

A PRIMER FOR APPLICATION OF THE CONCEPTS

PERSONAL AND FAMILY HEALTH ASSOCIATES

M. JOAN MUNLEY, Ed.D.
PATRICIA A. SAYERS, M.S.N.

i

Grateful acknowledgment is given to the following for permission:

Copyright ©1979 by Houghton Mifflin Co. Reprinted by permission from the *American Heritage Dictionary of the English Language*. Copyright ©1979 by Little Brown and Company. Reprinted by permission from *Concepts Formalization in Nursing: Process and Product*. Copyright ©1980 by McGraw-Hill Book Company. Reprinted by permission from *Nursing: Concepts of Practice*.

Artwork by Catherine S. Basch

Acknowledgments

A lot of living goes into creating a book. We thank those who lived with us while we worked: our families, friends and colleagues.

We thank Dr. Dorothea Orem for the inspiration her work provides.

Dr. Lois Evans cheered us on as she reviewed the manuscript and for this we are grateful.

A special thank you for editorial comments goes to Rita Roncher Weiner who gave generously of her skill, creativity and time.

This book was printed by Howard Press because Ken Rota believes in P.F.H. Assoc., Inc., a corporation wholly owned by nurses (us). We thank Howard Erny for his patience, endurance and good humor as he guided this publication through production.

M.J.M.
P.A.S.

Contents

ABOUT THIS BOOK AND US

We set out five years ago to put together a huge puzzle of related knowledge based on its structure and function. We wanted to do this so that we might have a means for integrating, or making whole, knowledge arranged in a hierarchy and relative to the Self-Care Deficit Theory of Nursing. The preface of this book tells the reader about our lofty goals. We now see these efforts as a lifetime of work.

Many books begin small and end large. The concept of this book began large and has grown small. As we shared our work with students, practitioners and clients we learned that the place to begin is with a demonstration of the fact that Self-Care Deficit Theory of Nursing is practical, useful and rewarding. We believe this primer meets these goals. Our next job is to continue to put together the remaining pieces of the puzzle.

M.J.M.
P.A.S.

Preface

Nursing is a science and an art requiring the application of concepts and theories. Advancements in the art of nursing are made as the science of nursing develops and is used in practice.

Over time, as practitioners and teachers of nursing, we have experienced the frustration of regarding our clients as whole beings, while the knowledge available for use in nursing is developed in individual disciplines. Further, nursing educators have for some time been struggling with the concept of the integrated curriculum. Again, knowledge is not integrated and the problem is addressed through bringing together pieces of individual disciplines in a course of study. The American Heritage Dictionary (1979) says that to integrate is to make whole by adding or bringing together parts. We argue that an assemblying of parts of the broad range of knowledge essential to nursing does not make it whole. This in fact, does not provide integrated knowledge, but assembles clusters of ideas which have potential for integration. For example, to bring together parts of Anthropology, Biology, Chemistry, Mathematics, Physics, Physiology, Sociology and others in isolation from a theoretical framework for nursing will not make an integrated body of knowledge, and therefore an integrated nursing curriculum. If integration is to take place, it must be done on the basis of theory, rather than a random assembly of parts of knowledge.

General Systems Theory (von Bertalanffy, 1968) provides a guide for integrating the various disciplines for use with nursing theory. It instructs the reader to consult the structure and function of related knowledge. Bringing together the bodies of related knowledge at the same level of complexity allows the integration of the knowledge. Ideas, as they are clustered together, form concepts. As one concept is put with another, a hierarchy of functional knowledge is created. Two ideas create a simply structured concept, three ideas a more complex structure, and on up a hierarchy of complexity, as each structure of knowledge takes in another idea. As the complexity of each structural concept grows, so does its functional capacity, or the ability to perform, act or "do". We argue

ix

on the basis of General Systems Theory for the *integration of related knowledge essential to nursing practice to take place at the same level of complexity.*

Human actions exemplify wholistic human functioning. For example, to pick up a pencil requires a harmonious integration of actions at the same level of complexity from the muscular, neurological and cognitive human systems among others. To write with the pencil requires a more highly structured or more complex integration of the functions of each system. The nurse can integrate knowledge from the related disciplines in a systematic way with the use of General Systems Theory and a theoretical model for nursing practice having a functional orientation. Dorothea Orem's General Theory of Nursing (1980) provides a focus enabling the nurse to describe and to measure the effectiveness of care according to a client's level of functioning.

When thinking of nursing as a science, the implication is that the service of nursing can be described, measured, and characterized as having predictable outcomes. The Self-Care Deficit Theory meets these criteria. This focus of nursing is to enhance the self-care capacity of clients, and to provide criteria for describing, measuring and predicting their functional activities. For example, the nurse can observe a client or a parent of a child as they learn self-care skill. The skill level, or self-care agency may be described and measured. The data from observations and measurements are assembled and then analyzed.

General Systems Theory and the Self-Care Deficit Theory of Nursing provide intellectual tools for integrating knowledge and measuring human functioning. We believe that the integration of knowledge as described here is theoretically sound and academically acceptable. We are eager to engage in the development of this line of thinking, and urge the reader to participate in professional dialogue regarding the ideas surrounding the integration of knowledge for nursing practice. This primer begins our effort toward these goals.

M. Joan Munley, Ed.D.
Patricia A. Sayers, M.S.N.

Introduction

The goal of this primer is to present the Self-Care Deficit Theory of Nursing (S.C.D.T.) in a way that will enable the reader to "think nursing". Theory systematically organizes knowledge, accepted principles and rules of procedure for application in a wide variety of circumstances.

Dorothea Orem's Self-Care Deficit Theory of Nursing provides a way of organizing nursing practice which, when mastered and implemented, gives form and structure to knowledge that describes and explains nursing (Orem, 1980,p.viii). The theory provides concepts which guide the selection of knowledge for use in nursing situations. It also explains the relation of the nurse to persons or to groups receiving nursing care.

This theoretical tool guides thinking for the practice of nursing and supplies a means for consumers and allied health professionals to understand nursing. Intended to be a handbook and an educational tool for teachers, students and practitioners of nursing, the text presents concepts of the Self-Care Deficit Theory of Nursing and practical ways of using the theory.

The objectives for the reader are to:
- **Recognize the concepts of the Self-Care Deficit Theory**
- **Define the recognized concepts**
- **Describe a way of thinking when applying the concept of the Self-Care Deficit Theory**
- **Identify practical uses of the concepts**

WHY USE THE SELF-CARE DEFICIT THEORY OF NURSING?

PART I

LINK

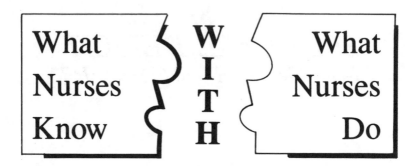

Self-Care Deficit Theory of Nursing meets a challenge for linking what the nurse knows with what the nurse does through guiding the selection and the use of knowledge.

Theories of Nursing

Theory provides a means for describing the boundaries of nursing and marks where nursing begins and ends. With intellectual tools for differentiating nursing from other health disciplines, practitioners have the ability to:

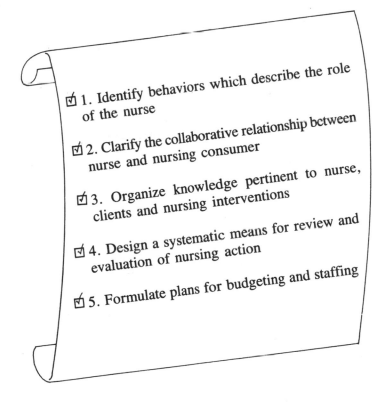

☑ 1. Identify behaviors which describe the role of the nurse

☑ 2. Clarify the collaborative relationship between nurse and nursing consumer

☑ 3. Organize knowledge pertinent to nurse, clients and nursing interventions

☑ 4. Design a systematic means for review and evaluation of nursing action

☑ 5. Formulate plans for budgeting and staffing

Theory Provides a Means for Creating a Role Description for Nurses

Concepts of the S.C.D.T. guide thinking for identification of behaviors expected of a nurse. Once nursing behaviors are identified it becomes possible to:

A. Clarify what nursing is and is not for health professionals and for society. Identification and clarification of nursing behaviors is essential for creating a role description for nursing.

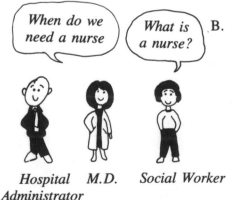

When do we need a nurse

What is a nurse?

Hospital Administrator *M.D.* *Social Worker*

B. Differentiate nursing requirements from a wide variety of demands for health care. This ability to discriminate nursing from other care disciplines promotes collaboration among health professionals and thereby maximizes the use of health care resources.

Theory Provides a Means For Describing
The Nursing Consumer

The Self-Care Deficit Theory describes nursing consumers as persons and/or support groups who lack the "ability to maintan continuously that amount and quality of self-care which is therapeutic in sustaining life and health, in recovering from disease or injury, or in coping with their effects" (Orem, 1980, p.7).

A clear description of the nursing consumer and what nursing is and is not guides consumers as they:

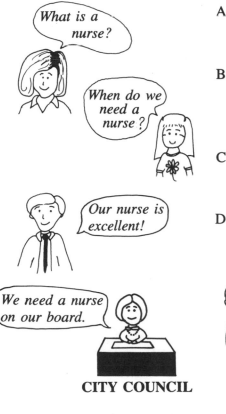

A. Identify role expectations and behaviors for both nurse and client

B. Recognize when nursing care is required for individuals, families and communities

C. Readily validate outcomes of nursing care

D. Recognize that quality health care for society requires nursing

Theory Provides a Means for Organizing Knowledge Pertinent to Nursing and To Nursing Consumers

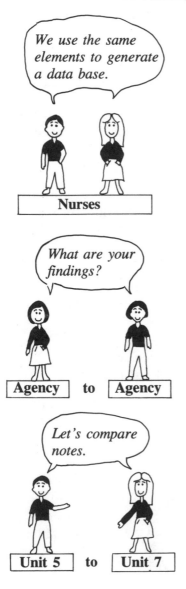

Self-Care Deficit Theory:

A. Provides guidelines for conducting a nursing assessment which, when used with groups of in-dividual clients will generate a comparable data base.

B. Clarifies communication and unites the efforts of nursing. With clear communications, nurses may join in solving nursing care problems.

C. Identifies, describes and organizes concepts pertinent to self-care deficits and nursing actions. Data related to these concepts can be stored systematically in a computer data bank and recalled for decision-making and care management.

A Quality of Care Assurance Program
Based in the S.C.D.T. of Nursing
Investigates the Relationship of Nursing
To Self-Care Outcomes

Self-Care Deficit Theory facilitates a systematic review and evaluation of nursing care through use of:

1) The language of the theory

2) A data base for decision making

3) Established outcome criteria

4) Standardize documentation procedures

**Nurse
Executive**

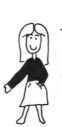

Quality Assurance activities have become more structured and meaningful since we adopted the S.C.D.T. in our Nursing Department.

**Chairperson of Quality
Assurance Committee**

Theory Guides the Formulation of Plans for Budgeting and Staffing on the Basis of Nursing Requirements

Measureable self-care deficits provide a base for determining essential nursing care. This care can be converted into kinds and amounts of nursing which translates into requirements for specific nursing skill levels and numbers of nurses. This data, gathered over time, provides a description of self-care deficits and identifies nursing requisites.

> Of course we want excellent nursing here; but if we are to increase your budget, I need concrete data supporting your recommendations! What are the client needs related to these requests? How will nursing use the funds?

HOSPITAL ADMINISTRATOR

Kind and Amount of Care Required	*minus* −	Self-Care Ability	*equals* =	Kind and Amount of Nursing Required

REVIEW I

WHY USE THE SELF-CARE DEFICIT THEORY OF NURSING?

1. Theory links what is known with what is done through guiding the selection and use of knowledge?

   True or False

2. Nursing behaviors may be identified by using the c_____ of the Self-Care Deficit Theory.

3. Persons and/or support groups who lack "ability to maintain continuously that amount and quality of self-care which is therapeutic in sustaining life and health, in recovering from disease or injury, or in coping with their effects" require n_____.

4. Use of a common: 1) language 2) data base 3) outcome criteria and 4) documentation method facilitates evaluation of nursing care.

   True or False

5.

Kind and Amount of Care Required	*minus* —	Self - Care Ability	*equals* =	K____ and A____ of N_____ R_____

PREPARING
FOR
THEORY-BASED NURSING
PRACTICE

PART II

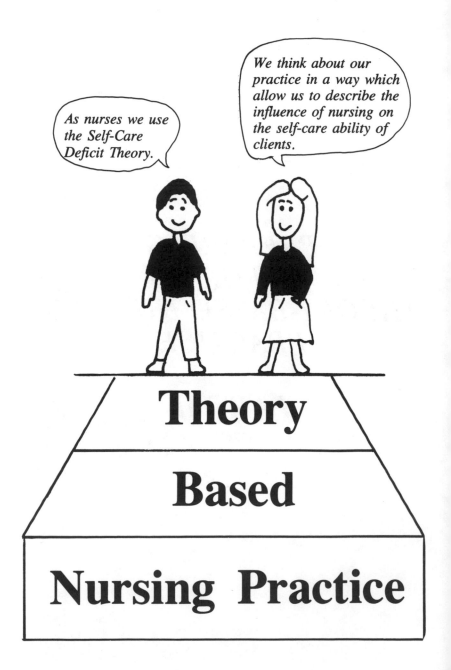

Concepts of Self-Care Deficit Theory Provide a Way of Thinking About Nursing Which:

A. Describes self-care abilities of clients

B. Guides assessment of the need for nursing

C. Describes nursing's contribution to changes in self-care ability.

D. Facilitates evaluation of nursing's contribution to changes in self-care ability.

E. Permits evaluation of the relationship of nursing to self-care outcomes.

Self-Care Deficit Theory Organizes Thought and Action for Practice

The theory guides the nurse to identify the:

1. **BOUNDARIES** of practice	Recognition of when nursing is required and where nursing begins and ends
2. **FOCUS** of practice	Humans with Self-Care Deficits
3. **GOALS** of practice	Establishing, maintaining and/or restoring self-care ability while contributing specialized knowledge and skill toward maintaining a therapeutic level of care.
4. **LANGUAGE** for practice	A consistent way of communicating with clients, peers and other professionals
5. **Evaluation** of care goals	To what degree were: a) care goals met b) self-care agency altered c) goals appropriate to self-care deficit

Self-Care Deficit Theory specifies: (1) boundaries, (2) focus, (3) goals (4) language and (5) evalution.

1 Boundaries of Practice

Self-Care Deficit Theory identifies when nursing is required.

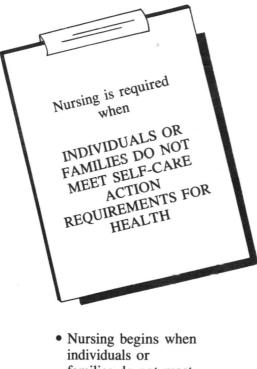

- Nursing begins when individuals or families do not meet self-care requirements.

- Nursing ends when individuals and families meet self-care requirements.

1 Boundaries of Practice

Nursing care is required when care actions of individuals and families do not meet requirements for self-care related to lack of:

P   •Attention span and vigilance

O

W   •Control of physical energy

E   •Control of body movements

R

   C   •Ability to reason

   O

   M   •Motivation for action

   P   •Decision-making skills

   O

   N   •Knowledge

   E   •Repertoire of skills

   N

   T   •Ability to order self-care actions

   S   •Ability to integrate self-care actions
into patterns of living

Adapted from
Nursing Development
Conference Group.
*Concept Formalization in
Nursing, Process and Product*, 2nd ed.,
edited by Dorothea E. Orem,
Little Brown and Company,
Boston, 1979

1 Boundaries of Practice

Nursing takes place wherever humans are found.

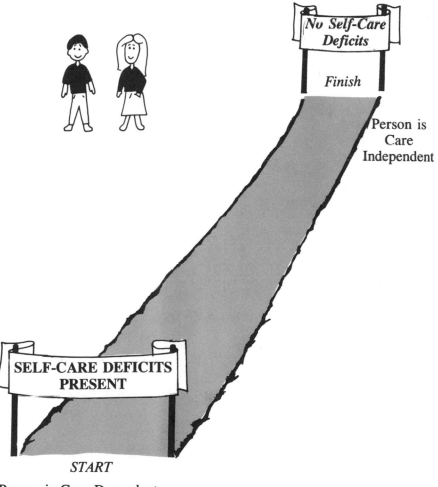

No Self-Care Deficits

Finish

Person is
Care
Independent

SELF-CARE DEFICITS
PRESENT

START

Person is Care Dependent

2 The Self-Care Deficit Theory Identifies
Nursing's Unique Focus

Humans require a variety of specialized services. Each service
has a unique focus.

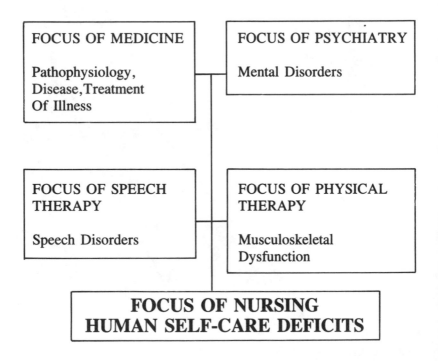

The focus of nursing is human self-care deficits.

3 A Goal of Practice

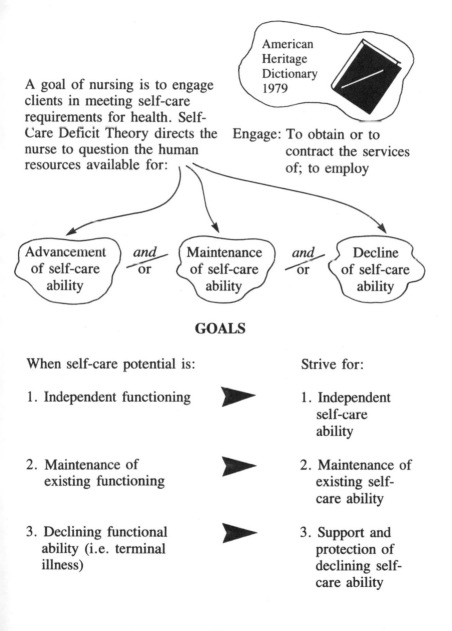

A goal of nursing is to engage clients in meeting self-care requirements for health. Self-Care Deficit Theory directs the nurse to question the human resources available for:

American Heritage Dictionary 1979

Engage: To obtain or to contract the services of; to employ

Advancement of self-care ability

and or

Maintenance of self-care ability

and or

Decline of self-care ability

GOALS

When self-care potential is:

1. Independent functioning

2. Maintenance of existing functioning

3. Declining functional ability (i.e. terminal illness)

Strive for:

1. Independent self-care ability

2. Maintenance of existing self-care ability

3. Support and protection of declining self-care ability

4 Language of the Self-Care Deficit Theory Provides a Vocabulary for Professionals, Peers, Consumers and Society

5. Evaluation of Care Goals

Goals which are determined to offset self-care deficit for the client are written in the nursing care plan; these goals become criteria for evaluation. A nurse questions to what degree were:

A. Care goals met.

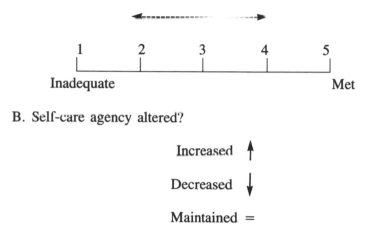

Inadequate   Met

B. Self-care agency altered?

Increased ↑

Decreased ↓

Maintained =

C. Care goals appropriate to self-care deficit?

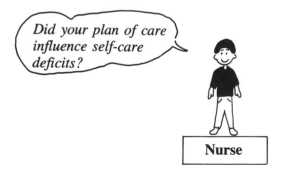

Did your plan of care influence self-care deficits?

Nurse

REVIEW II

PREPARING FOR THEORY-BASED NURSING PRACTICE

1. Nursing begins when individuals/families are not able to meet
   s_____-c _____ r _____.

2. Nursing ends when individuals and families are able to meet
   s_____-c _____r _____.

3. The focus of nursing is human s_____-c_____

   d_____.

4. Nursing may take place w _____humans are found.

VOCABULARY OF THE SELF-CARE DEFICIT THEORY

PART III

The vocabulary of the Self-Care Deficit Theory provides words and phrases which describe:

1. Self-Care Actions

2. Self-Care Deficits

3. Nursing Actions

4. Nurse-Client Relationships

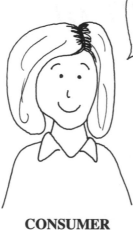

The language of the Self-Care Deficit Theory is useful and practical.

CONSUMER

Definition of self-care agency and dependent-care agency

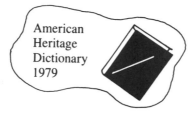

Self: the total being of one person
Agency: action, power, operation
Care: protection, supervision

Self + Care + Agency = Self-Care Agency
Or
A person's protective power

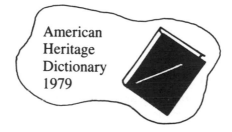

Dependent: unable to exist or function without
the aid or use of another
Agency: action, power, operation
Care: protection, supervision

Dependent + Care + Agency = Dependent-Care Agency
Or
A person's protective power for a dependent

Definition of Self-Care Agency and Dependent Care Agency

Q. What is self-care agency?
A. The ability of a person to engage in self-care

Q. What is dependent care agency?
A. The ability of a person to engage in infant care, child care or care of a dependent person

Q. Who has self-care agency?
A. Everyone!

Q. Who has dependent-care agency?
A. Individuals, families and other multiperson units responsible for the care of a dependent.

Q. Where is self-care and dependent care learned?
A. In social groups through human interaction and communication. (Orem, 1980, p. 28)

Every Person Possesses a Degree of Self-Care

Self-Care Agent

Self-Care Agents and Dependent-Care Agents

"We are responsible for our self-care and the care of our child."

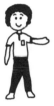

Self-Care Agent

"I'm solely responsible for my self-care"

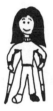

Self-Care Agent

"Right now I have some self-care deficits. My nurse is assisting me with care until I'm independent"

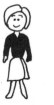 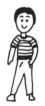

Self-Care Agent and Dependent Care Agent

Self-Care Agent

"We are responsible for our self-care and grandpa's too!"

Assessing self-care agency or dependent care agency requires questioning of:

a. Each individual's self-care ability

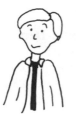

"I'm a solo self-care agent".

b. Dependent-care ability of a family or support group

- Family System

- Neighborhood Resources

- Significant Others

- Grandparents
  Teachers
  Camp Counselor
  etc.

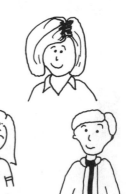

Assessment of self-care agency and dependent-care agency requires systematic evaluation of eight basic conditioning factors and ten power components.

Eight Basic Conditioning Factors

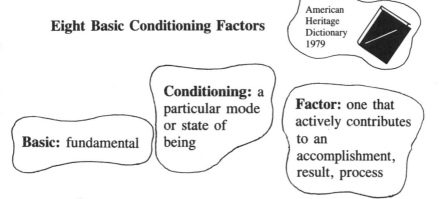

American Heritage Dictionary 1979

Conditioning: a particular mode or state of being

Factor: one that actively contributes to an accomplishment, result, process

Basic: fundamental

Baseline Data for Assessing the Individual

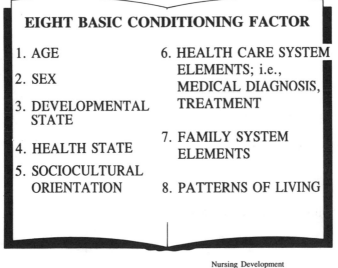

EIGHT BASIC CONDITIONING FACTOR

1. AGE
2. SEX
3. DEVELOPMENTAL STATE
4. HEALTH STATE
5. SOCIOCULTURAL ORIENTATION

6. HEALTH CARE SYSTEM ELEMENTS; i.e., MEDICAL DIAGNOSIS, TREATMENT

7. FAMILY SYSTEM ELEMENTS

8. PATTERNS OF LIVING

Nursing Development Conference Group. *Concept Formalization in Nursing, Process and Product,* 2nd ed., edited by Dorothea E. Orem, Little Brown and Company, Boston, 1979

Assessment of self-care agency and dependent care agency requires systematic evaluation of eight basic conditioning factors and ten power components.

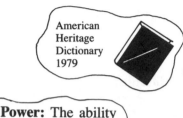

American Heritage Dictionary 1979

Power: The ability to act or perform effectively

Component: A simple part, or a relatively complex entity recorded as a part of a system, element constituent

- Attention span and vigilance

- Control of physical energy

- Control of body movement

- Ability to reason

- Motivation for action

- Decision-making skills

- Knowledge

- Repertoire of skills

- Ability to order self-care actions

- Ability to integrate self-care actions into patterns of living

Adapted from
Nursing Development
Conference Group.
*Concept Formalization in
Nursing, Process and Product*, 2nd ed.,
edited by Dorothea E. Orem,
Little Brown and Company,
Boston, 1979

REVIEW III

VOCABULARY OF THE SELF-CARE DEFICIT THEORY

1. Self-care agency is defined as the ability of a person to engage in self-care?

   True or False

2. Who has self-care agency?

3. A systematic assessment of self-care agency includes variables of the
   b _____ c _____ f _____.
   and p_____ c_____.

4. List eight basic conditioning factors influencing self-care agency.

   a.   e.

   b.   f.

   c.   g.

   d.   h.

5. List ten power components influencing self-care agency.

6. The person described as a dependent care agent performs the care given to a dependent person.

   True or False

7. When assessing self-care agency the dependent care-agent is assessed.

   True or False

SELF-CARE
DEFICITS

PART IV

Therapeutic Self-Care Demand

A self-care deficit exists when a person is unable to perform deliberate self-care acts necessary for health. A dependent-care deficit exists when a person who cares for another is unable to perform deliberate care acts necessary for the health of a dependent. Nursing is required when a self-care deficit exists in a person or in a dependent-care agent who cares for another person.

Self-care deficits and dependent-care deficits are determined by assessing the ability of care agents to meet three categories of care requisites contributing to therapeutic self-care demand.

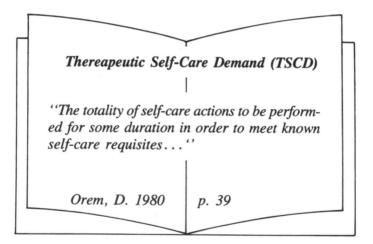

Thereapeutic Self-Care Demand (TSCD)

"The totality of self-care actions to be perform-ed for some duration in order to meet known self-care requisites..."

Orem, D. 1980 | *p. 39*

Self-Care Requisites

> *"Self-care requisites are expressions*
> *of the kinds of purposive self-care*
> *that individuals require"* *(Orem.1980,p.41).*

Behaviors which contribute to self-care requisites may be categorized.

The three categories of self-care requisites are:

Developmental
Self-Care
Requisites
(DSCR)

Universal
Self-Care
Requisites
(USCR)

Health Deviation
Self-Care
Requisites
(HDSCR)

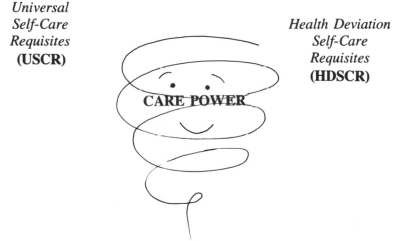

CARE POWER

USCR + DSCR + HDSCR=TSCD

Eight universal self-care requisites are required to promote and to preserve health in humans. The requisites are:

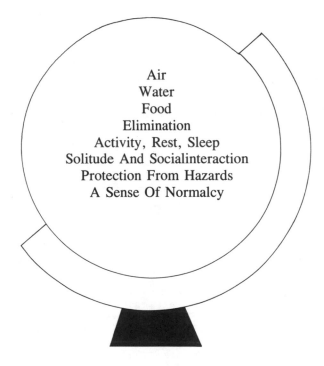

Air
Water
Food
Elimination
Activity, Rest, Sleep
Solitude And Socialinteraction
Protection From Hazards
A Sense Of Normalcy

UNIVERSAL SELF-CARE REQUISITES

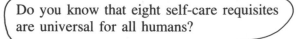

Do you know that eight self-care requisites are universal for all humans?

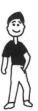

Developmental self-care requisites are met when:

A. An environment for the promotion of appropriate age and stage growth and development is provided.

AGE TO AGE   **STAGE TO STAGE**

One year old   Two years old   **Crawling   Walking**

B. Effects of injurious or potentially injurious events are prevented or minimized.

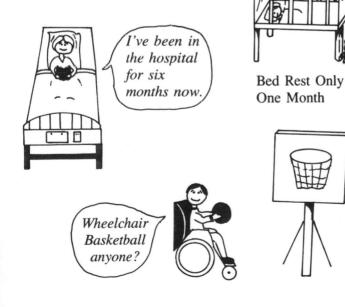

Health deviation self-care requisites exist in persons who

1. Become ill
2. Become injured
3. Have deficits or disabilities
4. Undergo medical diagnosis and/or treatment

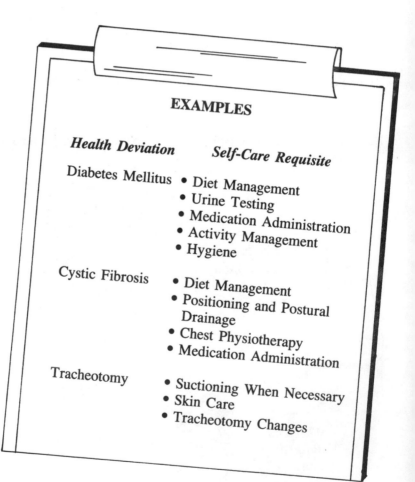

EXAMPLES

Health Deviation	Self-Care Requisite
Diabetes Mellitus	• Diet Management • Urine Testing • Medication Administration • Activity Management • Hygiene
Cystic Fibrosis	• Diet Management • Positioning and Postural Drainage • Chest Physiotherapy • Medication Administration
Tracheotomy	• Suctioning When Necessary • Skin Care • Tracheotomy Changes

Assessment of Self-Care Deficit and Dependent-Care Deficit

PHASE I.

When all care requisites are identified for individual clients and requisites are brought together. This collection of data is referred to as the therapeutic self-care demand.

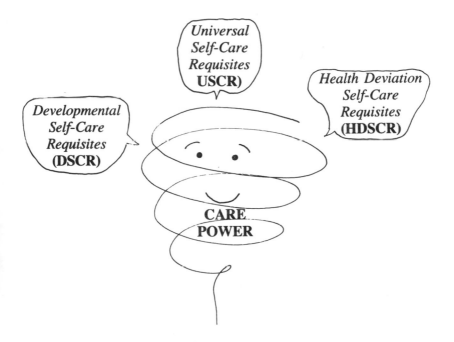

A nurse who has determined care requirements is prepared to proceed to the next phase of assessment of self-care deficit.

Move to the second phase
of self-care deficit assessment.

Assessment of self-care deficit and dependent-care deficit :

PHASE II

? Question the self-care agency or dependent-care agency available to a person for performing required self-care or dependent-care actions. Self-care and dependent-care agency is influenced by eight basic conditioning factors (B.C.F.) and ten Power Components.

Basic Conditioning Factors

1. Age
2. Sex
3. Developmental state
4. Health State
5. Sociocultural orientation
6. Health care systems elements
7. Family systems elements
8. Patterns of living

- 1. Attention span and vigilance
- 2. Control of physical energy
- 3. Control of body movement
- 4. Ability to reason
- 5. Motivation for action
- 6. Decision-making skills
- 7. Knowledge
- 8. Repertoire of skills
- 9. Ability to order self-care actions
- 10. Ability to integrate self-care actions into patterns of living

Nursing Development Conference Group. *Concept Formalization in Nursing, Process and Product,* 2nd ed., edited by Dorothea E. Orem, Little Brown and Company, Boston, 1979

Assessment of self-care deficit and dependent-care deficit:

When self-care agency (SCA) or dependent care agency (DCA) is less than therapeutic self-care demand (TSCD) there is respectively a self-care deficit (SCD) or a dependent-care deficit (DCD).

$$SCA <^* TSCD = SCD$$

$$DCA <^* TSCD = DCD$$

Therefore When:

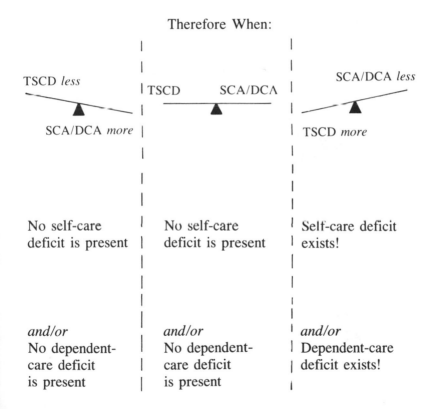

TSCD *less*

SCA/DCA *more*

TSCD   SCA/DCA

SCA/DCA *less*

TSCD *more*

No self-care deficit is present	No self-care deficit is present	Self-care deficit exists!
and/or No dependent-care deficit is present	*and/or* No dependent-care deficit is present	*and/or* Dependent-care deficit exists!

*Symbol for less than

Summary

When self-care agency (SCA) or dependent care agency (DCA) is less than therapeutic self-care demand (TSCD) there is a self-care deficit (SCD) or a dependent-care deficit (DCD) indicating a need for nurse agency (NA).

$$SCA < TSCD = SCD \rightarrow NA$$

$$DCA < TSCD = DSCD \rightarrow NA$$

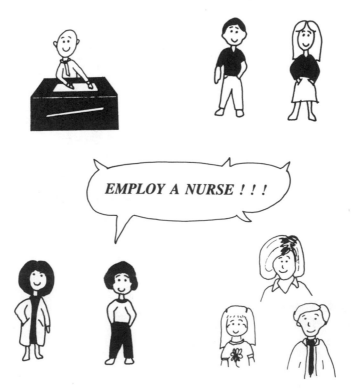

REVIEW IV

SELF-CARE DEFICITS

1. Self-care deficits are determined by assessing self-care ability to meet t_____ s_____- c_____ d_____.

2. List the Universal Self-Care Requisites

   a.   e.
   b.   f.
   c.   g.
   d.   h.

3. When age and stage growth and development are promoted and injurious life events are prevented or minimized the d____ s_____ -c_____ r_____ are met.

4. Self-care requisites associated with illness, injury, disability or medical treatments are called h_____ d _____ s _____ -c_____ r _____.

5. Describe the meaning of the following formula.

   SCA < TSCD = SCD → NA

NURSE AND CLIENT RELATIONSHIP

PART V

Nurse and client relationship

Self-Care Deficit Theory describes nurse/client relationships as being both:

1. Complementary
and
2. Contractural

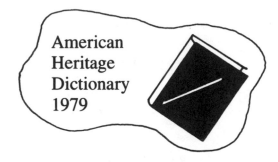

American
Heritage
Dictionary
1979

Complement: something that completes, makes up a whole

Complementary: forming or serving a complement (supplying mutual needs or lacks)

Contract: an agreement between two or more parties

Contractural: connected with or having the nature of a contract

Complementary

When self-care agency is limited by a deficit, the agency is complemented by the specialized knowledge and skill of a nurse. The care deficit is then supplemented and requirements for a therapeutic level of care are met.

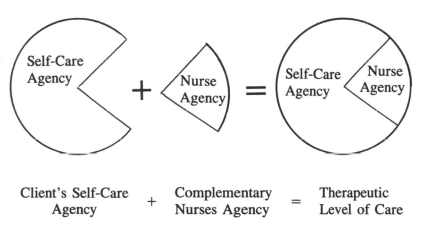

| Client's Self-Care Agency | + | Complementary Nurses Agency | = | Therapeutic Level of Care |

Complementary care completes, makes up a whole therapeutic level of care.

When nursing begins, deliberate action must be taken by client & nurse to develop a relationship. Each person actively negotiates to determine who will perform required care actions, when & for how long. Once decisions are agreed upon the product is a binding contract.

> **A nurse negotiates a binding contract with each client and complements the ability of each client**

Contract

Two questions must be answered when negotiating a contract between client and nurse:

1. What care is needed?

2. Who will provide the care?

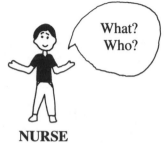

NURSE

A contract containing criteria for meeting care requisites is established when both nurse and client agree on the required care. An agreement is made to differentiate between the responsibility for care given by the nurse and the care given by the client. This contract is included in the care plan record.

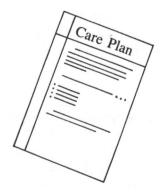

A contract contains criteria for measurement of care outcomes.

Comparing of the results of care (increased or decreased self-care agency) to establish criteria provides a measure of progress. The assumption is that each care giver, client and nurse, contribute to the progress of self-care according to the conditions of the contract.

> *I have a record of my care and its effectiveness.*

Nurse

As changes in self-care agency take place, the nurse revises the plan of care to complement the self-care agency of the client.

> *The progress made was remarkable. I'm ready for home care.*

Consumer

Contract

How will the contract between client and nurse be implemented?

How will individual responsibility for care be designated?

These two questions are answered through the process of contracting as follows:

PHASE I — CONTRACTING

A pool of information is established by the nurse. This data base includes:

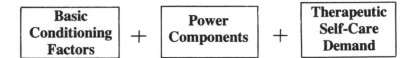

| Basic Conditioning Factors | + | Power Components | + | Therapeutic Self-Care Demand |

BASIC CONDITIONING FACTORS

- Age
- Sex
- Developmental state
- Health state

- Sociocultural orientation
- Health systems elements
- Family systems elements
- Patterns of living

Contract—Phase I

POWER COMPONENTS

- Attention span and vigilance

- Control of physical energy

- Control of body movement

- Ability to reason

- Motivation for action

- Decision-making skills

- Knowledge

- Repertoire of skills

- Ability to order self-care actions

- Ability to integrate self-care actions into patterns of living

THERAPEUTIC SELF-CARE DEMAND

1	2	3
Universal Self-Care Requisites	Developmental Self-Care Requisites	Health Deviation Self-Care Requisites
▼	▼	▼
• Air Water Food Elimination	• Age and stage throughout the life cycle	• Illness
• Activity, Rest, Sleep		• Disease
• Solitude, Soc.	• Environment	• Disability
• Normalcy Hazards		• Treatment, etc.

Phase II Contract

With this pool of information generated by assessment of basic conditioning factors, power components, and therapeutic self-care demands, the nurse is prepared to discuss, at the level of readiness of the client, the part each can play in restoring health. An agreement or contract is made between client and nurse so that the goals of care are met.

Care Plan Record
Nurse will instruct client
in Range of Motion
exercises.

Client will perform Range of
Motion exercises twice a day,
every day.

Evaluation of the contract

A contract containing measureable criteria for meeting care requisites is established between each nurse and client. An agreement is negotiated between the two which differentiates responsibility for providing care. The contract is included in the record of the care plan.

Once the caregiver, care measures, expected outcomes of self-care agency and care goals are designated, there is a structure for evaluation of care.

A structure is provided when:

1. **Each care measure is identified. The contribution of care given by the client or the nurse is recorded.**
2. **As changes in self-care agency take place, the nurse and client revise the plan of care to complement the self-care agency of the client.**

Evaluation of the contract requires the following questions:

1. **Does fulfillment of the contract meet care requisites?**
2. **To what degree do care measures provided by the client meet the goals of care?**
3. **Do care measures provided by the nurse meet the goals of care?**
4. **Did self-care agency increase, maintain or decline?**

1	2	3	4	5

REVIEW V

NURSE AND CLIENT RELATIONSHIP

1. Self-Care Deficit Theory describes the nurse-client relationship as being both **c** _____ **and c** _____.

2. The specialized knowledge and skill of a nurse **c** _____ the self-care agency of a client.

3. When nurse and client agree that care is required and they decide who will be responsible for providing this care a **c**_____ is established.

4.   Self-Care   Nurse   T_____

      Agency of + Agency = L_____

      Client   of C _____

5. As changes in self-care agency take place, **r** _____ are made in the plan of care.

NURSE AGENCY

PART VI

Nurse Agency

A nurse possesses specialized knowledge and skill for providing care. This ability to engage in nursing action is called nurse agency.

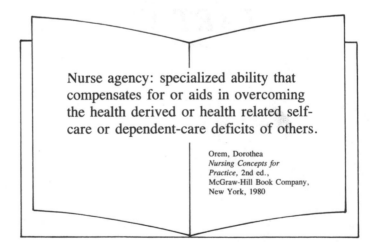

Nurse agency: power of one individual to provide for other individuals with health related self-care deficits; material and energy inputs essential for the self-maintenance and the health and well being of these others.

Nursing Development
Conference Group.
Concept Formalization in Nursing, Process and Product, 2nd ed., edited by Dorothea E. Orem, Little Brown and Company, Boston, 1979

Nurse agency: specialized ability that compensates for or aids in overcoming the health derived or health related self-care or dependent-care deficits of others.

Orem, Dorothea
Nursing Concepts for Practice, 2nd ed., McGraw-Hill Book Company, New York, 1980

Nurse Agency

AGENT One who acts for or as the
representative of another.

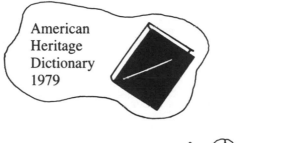

American
Heritage
Dictionary
1979

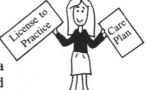

NURSE AGENT One who acts for a
client to provide specialized
nursing care.

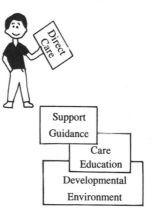

NURSE AGENCY is composed of
specialized knowledge and
skill, it is the
action and intellectual power
of the nurse.

Support
Guidance

Care
Education
Developmental
Environment

NURSE AGENCY PROVIDES

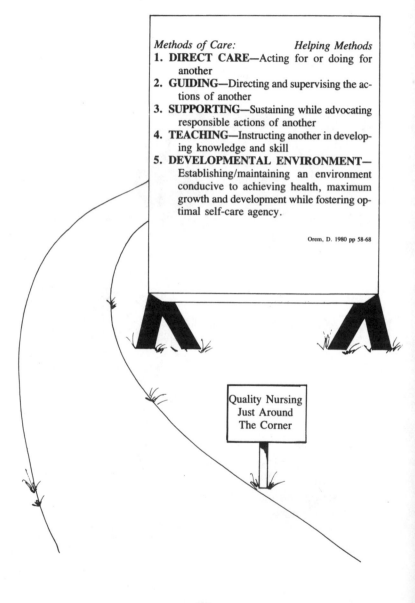

Methods of Care: *Helping Methods*
1. **DIRECT CARE**—Acting for or doing for another
2. **GUIDING**—Directing and supervising the actions of another
3. **SUPPORTING**—Sustaining while advocating responsible actions of another
4. **TEACHING**—Instructing another in developing knowledge and skill
5. **DEVELOPMENTAL ENVIRONMENT**—Establishing/maintaining an environment conducive to achieving health, maximum growth and development while fostering optimal self-care agency.

Orem, D. 1980 pp 58-68

Quality Nursing
Just Around
The Corner

How are both the quality and duration of care determined and described?

Nursing care complements the ability of a client to meet therapeutic self-care demands. This nurse agency provides the following systems of care:

Nursing System	Client State
Nurse agency is described as providing a:	When client is:
1. **Wholly compensatory nursing system**-nurse agency totally compensates for client self-care deficits	1. Totally care dependent Client unable to participate in self-care
2. **Partially compensatory nursing system**-nurse agency supplements client's limited self-care ability	2. Partially care dependent Client able to perform some but not all self-care actions
3. **Supportive-educative nursing system**-client performs self-care actions with support, teaching, guidance and developmental environment provided by the nurse	3. Able to be independent in self-care actions but needs assistance in learning self-care measures Orem, D. 1980 pp. 96–101

REVIEW VI

NURSE AGENCY

1. What methods of care are provided by nurse agency?

    a.   c.

    b.   d.

                                e.

2. Define the following terms:

    a. Wholly compensatory nursing system

    b. Partially compensatory nursing system

    c. Supportive-educative nursing system

3. The S.C.D.T. of Nursing describes a client as wholly compensatory.

    True or False

SELECTING THE SELF-CARE DEFICIT THEORY FOR PRACTICE

PART VII

What does a nurse need to know before adopting the Self-Care Deficit Theory of Nursing?

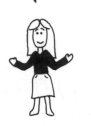

Are my personal beliefs in agreement with the principles of the S.C.D.T?

Using any theory of nursing requires that a nurse clarify his/her beliefs about humans, health and nursing. Effective use of the concepts of the theory relies upon consistency among personal beliefs and the principles of the theory.

In twenty-five words or less define the following terms according to your personal beliefs.

A. Humans _____
_____
_____

B. Health_____
_____
_____

C. Nursing _____
_____
_____

Self-Care Deficit Theory supports the beliefs that:

Humans are	• Rational • Capable of learning • Capable of deliberate action

Humans have	• Common needs
	• Continuous development
	• Requirements for care
	    a. Regulatory
	    b. Preventative

Health is	• A state of integrated structural and functional wholeness and soundness influenced by physical, psychological, interpersonal and social aspects of the individual.
Nursing	• Is a helping or assisting human service. • Clients may be persons, families, multiperson units, communities or special populations. • Is required when responsible persons are not able to perform necessary self-care practices. • Assures therapeutic levels of care. • Has as its focus self-care deficits. Orem, 1980

When the personal beliefs of each nurse agree with the principles of Self-Care Deficit Theory, she/he will benefit from using this theory as a tool for organizing practice. Assessment, planning, implementing and evaluation in this framework for nursing overcomes obstacles to communication and care giving for all who use the theory.

Once the decision to use the Self-Care Deficit Theory is made. How and when does the theory become operational?

The theory becomes operational as the nurse prepares for and then begins interaction with each client.

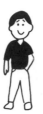

Hello, Mr. Jones. My name is Ed Topam. I am your primary nurse while you are in the hospital. Do you have any questions?

Nice to meet you Mr. Topam. Now I need help with a stomach problem.

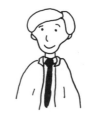

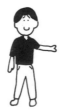

I read your health history. However, I will need more information from you. Let's plan to tour the unit now and meet later at 5 PM to plan your care.

The first meeting between nurse and client provides an opportunity for both to establish a complementary and a contractual relationship.

REVIEW VII

SELECTING THE SELF-CARE DEFICIT THEORY
FOR PRACTICE

1. Do your beliefs about humans agree with those of the S.C.D.T.?

   Yes or No

2. Do your beliefs abouts health agree with the S.C.D.T.?

   Yes or No

3. Are your beliefs about nursing congruent with the S.C.D.T.?

   Yes or No

4. When the personal beliefs of a nurse about humans and nursing conflict with S.C.D.T. nursing decisions and care management will be congruent with the model?

   Yes or No

5. The first meeting between nurse and client provides an opportunity for both to begin a complementary and a contractual relationship.

   True or False

IMPLEMENTATION OF THE SELF-CARE DEFICIT THEORY IN NURSING PRACTICE AND MANAGEMENT

PART VIII

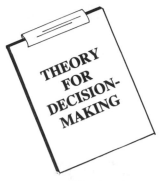
THEORY
FOR
DECISION-
MAKING

The S.C.D.T. provides a systematic way for nurses to make decisions as they give care.

Nurses are required to make decisions for the resolution of care problems. The nursing process, according to the S.C.D.T., involves three phases of problem solving:

Phase I Diagnosis and Prescription

A review of client data gives me information for diagnosis and prescription.

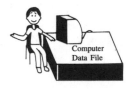
Computer
Data File

Phase II Designing and Planning

Mr.Doe, its 9:30 and I'd like to discuss your care as we agreed.

Phase III Production and Management

I did my intake and output.

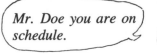

Mr. Doe you are on schedule.

Diagnosis and Prescription

Diagnosis is a determination of what can and should be done for the client now and in the future to meet the requirements of existing health care needs. When diagnosing self-care deficits the following variables are identified.

1. Care required
2. Ability of the client to perform self-care actions.
3. Client's self-care deficits.
4. Potential self-care deficits.

Through the processes of interview, inspection, observation and evaluation the client and care giver gather data for making a nursing diagnosis. Universal, developmental and health deviation self-care requisites, self-care agency and dependent-care agency are derived from the data.

Interview

Mr. Topam, I
need to know
how you have
been caring
for your
stomach
problems.

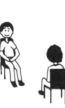

Inspection

Please take
a deep
breath.

Observation

This is how
I take my
medicine.

Evaluation

Now is the time to
evaluate the data we
have gathered

Nurse-Client

Nursing diagnosis: Phase I Continued

Nursing diagnoses are formulated whenever the following questions are answered.

QUESTION	DATA FOR FORMULATING AN ANSWER

1. *What is therapeutic self-care demand?*

1. USCR   DSCR   HDSCR
       T S C D

2. *What is client's self-care agency and/or dependent-care agency?*

2. Basic conditioning factors Age, sex, develomental state, health state, sociocultural orientation, health care elements, patterns of living and ten Power Components

3. *Does a self-care deficit exist? Does a dependent-care deficit exist?*

3. $SCA < TSCD = SCD \blacktriangleright NA$

   $DCA < TSCD = DCD \blacktriangleright NA$

4. *What variables contribute to*
   a. *a self-care deficit?*
   b. *a dependent-care deficit?*

4. Power components (Consult list of power components, see next page)

5. *Should a client be encouraged to participate in required care?*

5. Restriction? health state, sociocultural, resources, etc.

6. *What are realistic goals for client?*

6. Self-care agency Progression, maintenance, decline

Diagnosis and Prescription

Q. What is the format for writing a nursing diagnosis?

A. A standard format for writing a nursing diagnosis is not yet developed. One recommendation is to write a statement relating the:

1. Behaviors identifiable as essential to therapeutic self-care demand for health:
   a. Universal self-care requisites
   b. Developmental self-care requisites
   c. Health deviation self-care requisites

WITH

2. Identified power components influencing the deficit behavior. According to the Nursing Development Conference Group (1978) the power or capability to engage in self-care is influenced by:

A. Attention span and vigilance

B. Control of physical energy

C. Control of body movements

D. Ability to reason

E. Motivation for action

F. Decision making ability

G. Knowledge

H. Repertoire of skill

I. Ability to order self-care actions

J. Ability to integrate self-care actions into patterns of living

EXAMPLE: INABILITY TO REGULATE BLAND DIET RELATED TO LACK OF KNOWLEDGE

Diagnosis and Prescription

In Order to Prescribe:

1. Identify the care required. Determine whether the client has the ability to provide care. Mobilize complementary specialized skill.

2. Write a prescription that describes the care behaviors to be included in the self-care role and the behaviors included in the responsibility of the nurse agent.

Prescription for Care

Care Required:

1. _____
2. _____
3. _____

Role of the Client

1. _____
2. _____
3. _____

Role of the Nurse

1. _____
2. _____
3. _____

Diagnosis and Prescription

Data for formulating a nursing prescription is gathered from:

A. Specialized nursing knowledge relating to
Methods Procedures and actions

B. Values of the Client relating the care

C. Available Resources

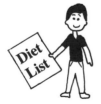

Nurse

Thank you for your diet suggestions. A vegetarian needs help with standardized menus.

Client

Designing and Planning

When the nurse diagnoses care requisites and prescribes nurse and client care roles the next step in the nursing process is to design a complementary system of care.

The nursing design provides a description of the complementary relationship between client and nurse. This includes:

A. Care actions   D. Outcome criteria

B. When   E. Methods

C. Sequence   F. Equipment

WHO	WHEN	Outcome Criteria
Who will do What care		Client will plan food menu for one week

SEQUENCE		
DATE	TIME	INTERVENTION
1-5-90	12:00 AM	After midnight the client is restricted from foods & fluids
1-5-90	6:00 AM	Nurse awakens client for his shower independently
1-5-90	9:30 AM	Nurse administers medications to client

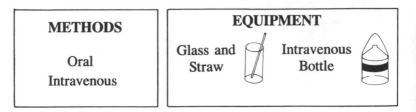

METHODS	EQUIPMENT
Oral Intravenous	Glass and Straw Intravenous Bottle

Designing and planning

Once a design for care is available a nurse needs to plan the support necessary to make each design a reality. A nursing plan addresses the:

- Number of nurses required

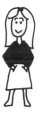 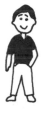

> *Mr. Jones is going to require 1 hour of your time tonight. Please schedule the staff so you can be available at 5pm.*

- Qualifications of nurses required

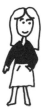 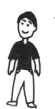

> *Teaching effectiveness will be a major factor in the success of Mr. Jones' care. Name the nurses who are prepared to teach with me.*

- Envirnomental conditions supportive to care goals

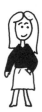 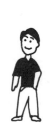

> *I need a quiet place to conduct Mr. Jones' teaching sessions.*

Production and management

In order to enter into a third phase of the nursing process, it is necessary to have

> 1. Diagnosed care requisites.
>
> 2. Prescribed care roles (Nurse and Client).
>
> 3. Designed a contractual and complementary system of care.
>
> 4. Planned for the nursing and environmental support to implement the design of care.

Once the plan is produced it is then possible to begin caring behaviors toward completing the proposed plan.

> *Production of care takes place as the plan is implemented through nursing modes of (1) direct care, (2) support, (3) guidance, (4) education and (5) providing for a developmental environment.*

> # NURSING IN ACTION
> # PRODUCTION IS
> # IMPLEMENTATION

Production and management Phase III continued

Management takes place throughout care production; it requires ongoing evaluation of care outcomes. A nurse evaluates care outcomes in terms of change in self-care requisites and self-care agency. One questions whether the self-care requisites and the self-care agency have:

1. Increased

2. Decreased

3. Remained the same

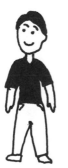

> *Client care requisites have declined. The client is now able to function more independently as a self-care agent.*

Care management requires continuing analysis of diagnosis, prescription, design, plan and production.

REVIEW VIII

IMPLEMENTATION OF THE SELF-CARE DEFICIT THEORY OF NURSING PRACTICE AND MANAGEMENT

1. Nursing process, according to the S.C.D.T., involves three phases of problem solving. These phases are:

   a) D _____ and p _____

   b) D _____ and p _____

   c) P _____ and m _____

2. Describe: a) Nursing diagnosis and prescription

   b) Nursing design and plan

   c) Nursing production and management

DOCUMENTATION

PART IX

The following variables are essential components of a recording system for S.C.D.T.:

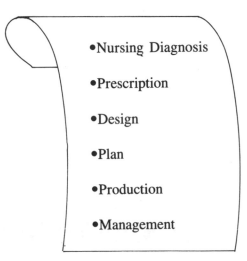

- Nursing Diagnosis
- Prescription
- Design
- Plan
- Production
- Management

Behaviors and events influencing nurse and client interactions generate a need for the following records:

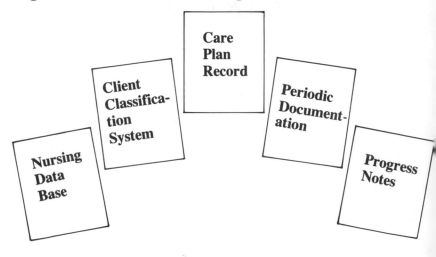

Care Plan Record

Client Classification System

Periodic Documentation

Nursing Data Base

Progress Notes

Documenting a Nursing Data Base

Information essential to a nursing history forms a record which guides the nurse in assessing and recording: 1) universal, 2) developmental, 3) health deviation self-care requisites, and 5) self-care agency.

NURSING HISTORY	Client Name
Basic Conditioning Factors Age _____Sex _____Developmental State _____ _____Health State _____ Sociocultural Orientation _____ Health Care System Elements _____ Family System Elements _____ Patterns of living _____ _____	
Therapuetic Self-Care Demand	Nursing Dx.
Universal Self-Care Requisites	
Developmental Self-Care Requisites	
Health Deviation Self-Care Requisites	

Documenting Nursing Diagnosis

Nursing care is continuous and begins with a nursing history. The first nursing diagnoses are written in the nursing history along with the data supporting these conclusions. Thereafter, nursing diagnoses are written in the periodic documentation of care.

NURSING HISTORY	Client Name *Mr. Jones*
(Data Base) Basic Conditioning Factors Age ___42___ Sex _Male_ Developmental State _Functionally_ _Independent_ Health State _____ Sociocultural Orientation _____ Health Care System Elements _____ Family System Elements _____ Patterns of living _____ _____	

Therapuetic Self-Care Demand	Nursing Dx.
Universal Self-Care Requisites *Food: Client states lack of knowledge regarding bland diet; dependent in food selection and food preparation.*	*Inability to regulate bland diet related to lack of knowledge*
Developmental Self-Care Requisites	
Health Deviation Self-Care Requisites	

Documenting Nursing Prescription

Prescriptions for nursing care and self-care are formulated to supplement self-care deficits noted in the nursing diagnosis. These prescriptions are documented in the record of the nursing care plan.

NURSING CARE PLAN RECORD			Clients Name
Date	Nursing Dx.	Goal	Interventions
1-5-90	Inabilty to regulate bland diet related to lack of knowledge	Client and wife will •define a bland diet •plan a menu for one week •list preparation concerns •describe integration of diet into life style	1. Nurse to teach protocol for bland diet- Vegetarian 1/6/90 4:00 PM 2. Review diet with family members...

Documenting Nursing Design

Individualized care requires a record of each nursing design: this records includes: 1) specific care actions, 2) sequences of care, 3) outcome criteria and 4) methods and equipment appropriate to each design. This written design is added to each nursing care plan.

Nursing Care Plan Record		Clients Name Mr. Jones	
Date	Nursing Dx.	Goal	Interventions
1-5-90	Inability to regulate bland diet related to lack of knowledge	Client and wife will •define a bland diet by 1/7/90 •plan food menu for one week 1/9/90 •list preparation concerns 1/10/90	Nurse to teach protocol for bland diet-vegetarian 1/6/90 2:00 pm, 1/7/90 5:00 pm, 1/8/90 2:00 pm, 1/9/90 5:00 pm, 1/10/90 2:00 pm Review diet preparation in ADL kitchen with client and family 1/8/90 5:00 pm, 1/10/90 5:00 pm

Documenting Nursing Plans For Both Individuals and Groups

When nursing diagnosis, care prescriptions and nursing designs are complete, the next step is to question the total amount and kind of nursing required for each client. Provision of a therapeutic level of care must be assured. This includes:

- NUMBERS OF NURSES

- QUALIFICATIONS OF NURSE

- ENVIRONMENT FOR NURSING

When using S.C.D.T., client care needs are identified and then classified according to:

A) Universal self-care requisites

B) Developmental self-care requisites

C) Health deviation self-care requisites

Classified care needs are then scaled according to the intensity of nursing care required.

SCA Adequate   SCA Inadequate
```
          1     2     3     4     5
          |_____|_____|_____|_____|
```

Scale for Classicication of Self-Care Agency

	SCA ADEQUATE			SCA INADEQUATE	
AIR	1	2	3	4	5
WATER FOOD	1	2	3	4	5
ELIMINATION	1	2	3	4	5
ACTIVITY, REST, SLEEP	1	2	3	4	5
SOLITUDE AND SOCIAL INTERACTION	1	2	3	4	5
PROTECTION FROM HAZARDS	1	2	3	4	5
SENSE OF NORMALCY	1	2	3	4	5
HEALTH DEVIATION CARE MANAGE.	1	2	3	4	5
DEVELOPMENTAL CARE MANAGEMENT	1	2	3	4	5

Adapted from Orem, D., *Nursing: Concepts of Practice*, 2nd Ed. McGraw-Hill, N.Y. 1980 pp. 39–53

Nursing requirements for supplementing SCA need to be specified in terms of: direct care, teaching, support, guidance and development environment.

Nursing Systems of Care

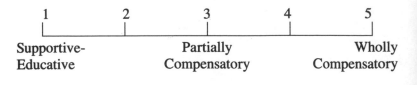

1	2	3	4	5
Supportive-Educative		Partially Compensatory		Wholly Compensatory

Documenting the kinds and amounts of nursing planned for both individuals and groups

Nursing plans framed in the S.C.D.T. specify kinds and amounts of nursing required for each client. Nursing is classified into: direct care, teaching, support, guidance and provision of a developmental environment. When the nursing hours for each classification of care are totalled and documented nursing coordinators, managers and executives are informed of the quantity of nursing to be provided. These persons are then able to make decisions for staffing and scheduling the care of clients on the basis of nursing requirements, as opposed to the size of the client population.

For example:

Self-Care Classification	Client Name *Mr. Jones*				
Air	(1)	2	3	4	5
Water and Food	1	2	(3)	4	5
Elimination	(1)	2	3	4	5
Etc.	(1)	2	3	4	5

Nursing System of Care	Client Name: *Mr. Jones*			
	Supportive Educative	Partially Compensatory		Wholly Compensatory
Air	(1)	2	3	4	5
Water and Food	1	2	(3)	4	5
Elimination	(1)	2	3	4	5
Etc.	(1)	2	3	4	5

Documenting the kinds and amounts of nursing planned for both individuals and groups

Examples continued:

Nursing Methods		Client Name: *Mr. Jones*
Time	**Method**	**Allotment**
Day	Direct Care	1 Nursing Hour
	Teaching	1 Nursing Hour
Evening	Direct Care	1 Nursing Hour
	Teaching	1 Nursing Hour
Night	Direct Care	1 Nursing Hour

Total Nursing Hours for a 24 Hour Period=5 Hours

Fee for service: Nursing Hours __5__ ×Hourly Rate=
24 Hour Fee For Service

Unit Requirements For Nursing

35 clients/Unit B
1. Total Nursing Hours for Unit B=56 Nursing Hours
2. 56 Nursing Hours÷8 HourShift=7 Nurses
3. Therefore Unit B requires the services of 7 Nurses

16 hrs. of Direct Care
18 hrs. of Teaching
12 hrs. of Guidance/Support
10 hrs. of Developmental Environment
56 hrs. of Nursing Care

Documenting Nursing Production

Nursing documentation includes notes on the production of nursing care. Periodic documentation includes significant events relevant to change in care requisites. When change in prescription and design of nursing is updated remember to question the need for change in the nursing care plan.

NURSING NOTES		Client's Name Mr. Jones
Date/Time	Nursing Dx.	Notation
1/6/90 5:00 PM	Inability to regulate bland diet related to lack of knowledge	Client states his work will involve travel for the next 9 months; he will be eating in restaurants much of the time. Focus for planning addresses selection of a bland diet from restaurant menus. Client described a bland diet after reviewing section one of the teaching protocol. Will continue to teach, to support and to guide client according to care plan. E.T.

Documenting Nursing Management

Change in self-care ability shifts the need for nursing; requirements may increase or decrease. As the kind and amount of nursing is altered, adjustment in the nursing system of care takes place. Shifts of nursing system become reciprocal indicators of change in self-care agency of clients.

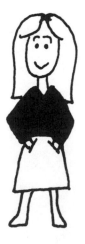

Mr. Jones can describe a bland diet, plan his own menus and prepare foods according to diet requirements. Now I am providing a supportive-educative nursing system.

Documenting Nursing Management

Evaluation of change in the self-care abilities of each client is documented by the nurse in her/his notes on care—or in inter-disciplinary progress notes.

Nursing Documentation or Progress Notes		Client Mr.Jones
Date/ Time	Nursing Dx	Summary
1/10/90 5:00 PM	Inability to regulate bland diet related to lack of knowledge	Client demonstrates appropriate selection of foods. Refer to the notations of the teaching protocol. Will supervise client's dietary management during remainder of hospitalization. E.T.

Documentation Ends

Once a nursing staff establishes a standardized record for all nursing, it is used throughout the sequence of care from admission to discharge. Ongoing assessment, planning, implementation and evaluation of care is recorded until the contract for care is fulfilled or the client leaves the service setting with provisions made for the continuity of care. When the conditions of a contract are met and the records are complete nursing is no longer required.

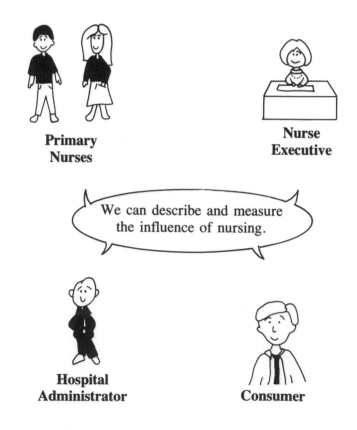

Primary Nurses

Nurse Executive

We can describe and measure the influence of nursing.

Hospital Administrator

Consumer

REVIEW IX

DOCUMENTATION

1. A nursing history is a record which guides the nurse in assessing and recording: 1) universal, 2) developmental, 3) health deviation self-care requisites and self-care and dependent care agency.

   True or False

2. Nursing diagnoses are derived from data found in a nursing data base.

   True or False

3. Prescriptions designate the care actions required.

   True or False

4. In order to fulfill the contract made between nurse and client a design for care including 1) care actions, 2) sequence of care, 3) outcome criteria and 4) methods and equipment must be completed.

   True or False

5. A plan for caring requires the support necessary to make the design a reality and includes n_____ of nurses q _____ of nurses and e _____ for nurses.

IMPLEMENTING THE SELF-CARE DEFICIT THEORY OF NURSING IN A PRACTICE SETTING

PART X

**Translating Nursing Theory into Practice
Requires:**

- **Committement** to nursing as a profession

- Determination of agency and/or practice **philosophy, goals and objectives**

- Selection of a **nursing theory** congruent with the determined philosophy, goals and objectives.

- Integration of the selected theoretical model into **orientation, inservice and continuing education programs.**

- Development of role descriptions and care protocols in keeping with the model.

- Use of concepts of the model to devise a **documentation system.**

- Use of the theory when providing nursing for **client care**

- Use of the concepts of the model to develop **quality assurance** activity.

- Communication among professionals concerning implementation, evaluation and development of the model—**Networking.**

- Clinical **research** and contribution to theory development.

Commitment

Members of the nursing staff must believe the following:

1. Nursing provides a unique contribution to client health care.

2. Nursing's contribution to care can be described and measured.

Philosophy, goals and objectives

A shift from technical to theory-based nursing practice requires
that members of a nursing system collaborate in determining
a collective philosophy which may be translated into goals and
objectives for practice.

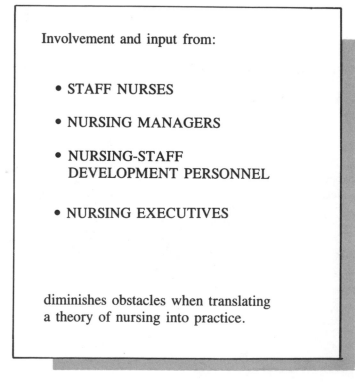

Involvement and input from:

- STAFF NURSES

- NURSING MANAGERS

- NURSING-STAFF
  DEVELOPMENT PERSONNEL

- NURSING EXECUTIVES

diminishes obstacles when translating
a theory of nursing into practice.

Nursing Theory

Assessment of nursing models to question their agreement with a group's philosophy of nursing, goals and objectives for care is the next step in implementing theory based nursing practice.

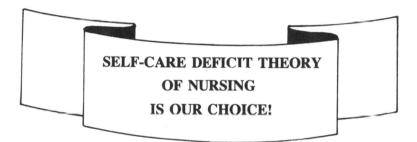

SELF-CARE DEFICIT THEORY
OF NURSING
IS OUR CHOICE!

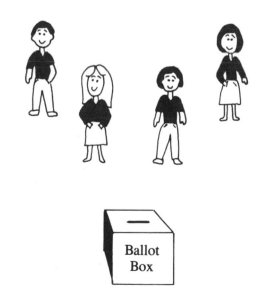

Ballot
Box

Orientation, inservice and continuing education

Orientation programs, as well as inservice and continuing education offerings, must utilize the concepts of the Self-Care Deficit Theory.

Orientation Content Outline

Week 1   Introduction of concepts
6 Hrs.   SCDT

Week 2   Care Management
2 Hr.   and decision making
             based on SCDT

Week 3   Unit management
2 Hr.   based on SCDT

Annual Conference

Self-Care Deficit Theory
of Nursing

University of America
Washington, D.C.

Inservice Announcement

"Promoting Self-Care
Agency of the School
Age Child"

Case study presentation
by Ms. Johnson R.N.

Main Auditorium
10:30-11:30 a.m.

Open admission

Documentation

Concepts of a nursing theory provide a guide for organizing a record keeping system congruent with the theory.

Use of committees made up of:

1. Staff nurses

2. Nurse Managers

3. Nurse-Staff development personel

4. Nurse executives

Maximizes communication, and personal investment in success of the record keeping system.

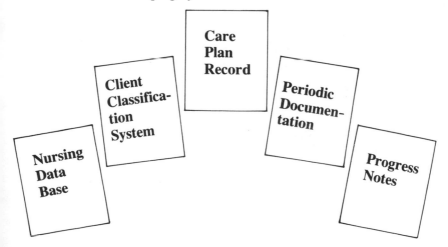

Client care

When plans, actions and evaluation of nursing and self-care are based on the concepts of the Self- Care Deficit Theory, theory based nursing is launched.

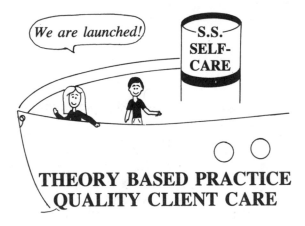

Quality Assurance

S.C.D.T. provides a structure for the systematic review and evaluation of nursing's contribution to the goals planned for clients. This evaluation monitors quality assurance and enables the nursing department of an agency to meet the Joint Commission for the Association of Hospital's departmental criteria for accreditation.

Examples of application of the S.C.D.T. in nursing quality assurance activity include:

1) Observation validating the fulfillment of self-care goals.

2) Client/family interviews and questionnaires describing the complementary and the contractual nature of nursing systems of care.

3) Audits of documentation systems verifying the use of the nursing process as described by Orem.

4) Questioning the need for nursing and the classification of care into nursing systems. These systems become tools for planning, implementing, and evaluating nursing care requirements.

5) Standards of care and outcome criteria based on the S.C.D.T.

Networking

Networks of colleagues committed to the development and to the dissemination of the Self-Care Deficit Theory of Nursing are centered in colleges, schools of nursing and health care agencies. Nurses in education, practice and research are collaborating toward the refinement and testing of clinical tools, mathematical formulas for computing relationships among self-care agency, nurse agency and self-care deficits. Development of computer software is one of many innovations underway.

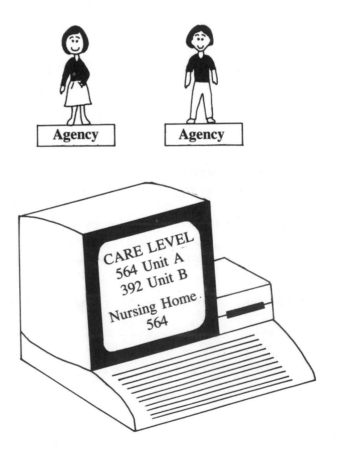

Research

The systematic use of S.C.D.T. of Nursing creates a field for clinical research. The concepts of the theory provide structure for describing, measuring and testing relationships among self-care, self-care deficits and nursing systems.

SELF-CARE DEFICIT THEORY
OF NURSING:

A GENERAL THEORY

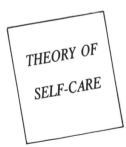

THEORY OF

SELF-CARE

THEORY OF

SELF-CARE

DEFICIT

THEORY OF

NURSING

SYSTEMS

REVIEW X

IMPLEMENTING THE SELF-CARE DEFICIT THEORY OF NURSING IN A PRACTICE SETTING

1. A shift from technical to theory based practice requires collaboration among members of a nursing system for determination of collective philosophy which may be translated into goals and objectives for practice.

   True or False

2. Collaboration among nursing staff, managers, educators and executives is required for theory based nursing.

   True or False

3. Concepts of a nursing theory provide a guide for organizing a record keeping system congruent with theory based practice.

   True or False

4. Nurses in education, practice and research are collaborating in the further development and refinement of the Self-Care Deficit Theory.

   True or False

5. Systematic use of the S.C.D.T. of Nursing creates a field for clinical research.

   True or False.

Review Responses

I. Why Use The Self-Care Deficit Theory of Nursing, Page 9
1. True 2. Concepts 3. Nursing 4. True 5. Kinds and Amount of Nursing

II. Preparing For Theory-Based Nursing Practice, Page 22
1. Self-care requirements 2. Self-care requirements 3. Self-care deficits 4. Wherever

III. Vocabulary Of The Self-Care Deficit Theory, Page 31
1. True 2. Everyone 3. Basic conditioning factors and Power components 4. Age, sex, developmental state, health state, sociocultural orientation, health care systems elements, family system elements and patterns of living. 5. Attention span and vigilance, control of physical energy, control of body movements, ability to reason, motivation for action, decision-making skills, knowledge, repertoire of skills, ability to order self-care action, and ability to integrate self-care actions into patterns of living. 6. True. 7. True

IV. Self-Care Deficits, Page 43
1. Therapeutic self-care demand 2. Air, water, food, elimination, activity, rest, sleep, solitude and social interaction, protection from hazards and a sense of normalcy 3. Developmental self-care requisites 4. Health deviation self-care requisites 5. When self-care agency is less than therapeutic self-care demand a self-care deficit exists requiring nurse agency.

V. Nurse And Client Relationship, Page 54
1. Contractual and complementary 2. Complements 3. Contract 4. Therapeutic level of care 5. Revise

VI. Nurse Agency, Page 60
1. Direct care, teaching, support, guidance and provision for a developmental environment 2a. Whilly compensatory nursing system-nurse agency totally compensates for client self-care deficits while a client is totally care dependent. b. par-

tially compensatory nursing system of care-nurse agency suplmenets client's limited self-care ability while a client performs some but not all self-care actions. c. Supportive-educative nursing system-nurse agency provides support, teaching, guidance and a developmental cnvironment while a client performs self-care actions required. 3. False. Wholly compensatory refers to a nursing system. When a wholly compensatory nursing system is implemented the client can be described as totally care dependent.

VII. Selecting The Self-Care Deficit Theory For Practice, Page 65

1-3. Answer according to your beliefs 4. No 5. True

VIII. Implementation Of The Self-Care Deficit Theory In Nursing Practice and Management, Page 78

1a. Diagnosis and prescription b. Designing and planning c. Production and management. 2 a. Diagnosis is a determination of what can and should be done for the health of each client. Prescription identifies the care and care roles to be carried out by both the nurse and the client. b. Nursing design provides a description of the complementary relationship between client and nurse including specific care actions, time, sequence, outcome criteria, methods and equipment. Nursing plan addresses the numbers of nurses, qualifications of nurses and environment for nursing required to implement the nurse and client contract. Nursing production refers to the process of implement the nurse and client contract. Management reflects ongoing analysis of diagnosis, prescription, design and production.

IX. Documentation Page 93

1. True 2. True 3. True 4. True 5. Number, qualifications and environment

X. Implementing The Self-Care Deficit Theory Of Nursing In A Practice Setting, Page 106

1. True 2. True 3. True 4. True 5. True

Bibliography

1. Morris, W., *The American Heritage Dictionary of the English Language*. Boston: Houghton Mifflin Co., 1979

2. Nursing Development Conference Group, *Concept Formalization In Nursing: Process And Product* (2nd Ed.). Boston: Little, Brown and Company, 1979

3. Orem, D.E., *Nursing: Concepts Of Practice* (2nd Ed.). New York, McGraw-Hill, 1980

Readings

1. Bennett, J.G. (Guest Ed.) "Symposium on the self-care concept of nursing". *Nursing Clinics Of North America*, 1980, 15, 129–217.

2. Chinn, P.L. and Jacobs, M.K. *Theory And Nursing A Systematic Assessment* St. Louis: C.V. Mosby, 1983

3. Fawcett, Jr. *Analysis And Evaluation Of Conceptual Models In Nursing* Philadelphia: F.A. Davis, 1984

4. Riehl, J.P. and Roy, C. *Conceptual Models For Nursing Practice* (2nd Ed.). New York: Appleton-Century-Crofts, 1980